# YOUR KNOWLEDGE HAS VALUE

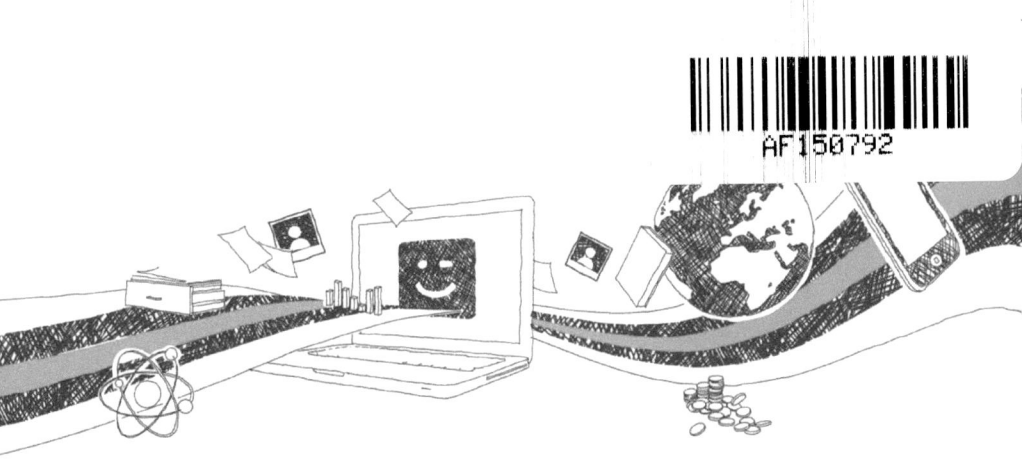

- We will publish your bachelor's and master's thesis, essays and papers

- Your own eBook and book - sold worldwide in all relevant shops

- Earn money with each sale

Upload your text at www.GRIN.com
and publish for free

**Bibliographic information published by the German National Library:**

The German National Library lists this publication in the National Bibliography; detailed bibliographic data are available on the Internet at http://dnb.dnb.de .

**Imprint:**

Copyright © 2015 GRIN Verlag
Print and binding: Books on Demand GmbH, Norderstedt Germany
ISBN: 9783668088382

**This book at GRIN:**

https://www.grin.com/document/310038

Thufail Korankulangara

# Enabling Factors for Neighbourhood Network in Palliative Care (NNPC). An Exploratory Study in Kozhikode District, Kerala

GRIN Verlag

**GRIN - Your knowledge has value**

Since its foundation in 1998, GRIN has specialized in publishing academic texts by students, college teachers and other academics as e-book and printed book. The website www.grin.com is an ideal platform for presenting term papers, final papers, scientific essays, dissertations and specialist books.

**Visit us on the internet:**

http://www.grin.com/

http://www.facebook.com/grincom

http://www.twitter.com/grin_com

# Enabling factors for Neighbourhood Network in Palliative Care (NNPC); An Exploratory study in Kozhikode district, Kerala.

A dissertation submitted during 2015 to the University of Hyderabad in partial fulfilment of the award of a Master degree in Public Health

Submitted by,

Thufail Korankulangara

School of Medical Sciences

University of Hyderabad

(P.O.) Central University, Gachibowli

Hyderabad - 500 046

Telangana

India

# CONTENTS

## ACKNOWLEDGEMENTS

First I would like to thank the School of Medical sciences for giving me an opportunity and necessary guidance to complete this project.

I thank my guide and supervisor Dr Katta Ajitha and my co-supervisor Mr. Nanda Kishore Kannuri for providing needed inputs for the completion of project.

And I must thank lot of people who have contributed many things for doing and completing this project work. Thank you all for your help!

# ABSTRACT

**Introduction:** This study attempts to explore the enabling factors for Neighbourhood Network in Palliative Care (NNPC, in Kozhikode district, Kerala India.). **Method:** fifteen participants were selected by purposive snowball sampling. This includes volunteers, socio-political leaders and NNPC leaders. The participants were interviewed and the entire conversation was audio recorded. The interview transcripts were analysed using the thematic analysis techniques.     **Results:** The data analysis revealed eight themes such as socio cultural factors, health pattern and demographic factors, behavioural and environmental factors, organizational factors, administrative factors, community Participation/ ownership and other factors and subsequent subthemes. All these themes and sub-themes showed different types of factors that enabled a successful community owned palliative care program. **Conclusions:** The enabling factors which are explored through this study categorized into eight types.

**Key words:** NNPC, community owned program, palliative care and enabling factors

# INTRODUCTION

Palliative care is a specialized area of modern medicine, which focuses on relieving and preventing the suffering of patients. It includes the care of patient and family, pain and symptoms management, disease modifying treatments, psychological, spiritual and social support and bereavement support. Theoretically palliative care goes well beyond the biomedical model of health by its 'holistic approach' of care.

In India, 5.4 million people estimated to be need of palliative care. It includes cancer patients, elder people, people who are at end stage of systemic disease, AIDS etc. out of 5.4 million people less than 2% of people only getting service of palliative care in India. It means that, in India there should be a mechanism which can serve the need of palliative care to those who needed. Modern medical system is more concerned about the curative aspects of diseases. At the same time the numbers of people who don't have any hope on cure of their diseases are increasing day by day like terminally ill, long term diseased and disabled persons.

In Kerala, palliative care activities are comparatively strong. In a study done in Malappuram District of Kerala it was found that around 40% of those people who are dying would have benefited from applying the principles of palliative care in their management. In Kerala, with a population of 32 million and a crude death rate of 6.3 (Reference: Census 2001) around 80,000 dying patients and their families would be benefited each year. To this if we add the number of people living for years with chronic conditions the total number will be much more.

The palliative care services delivering in Kerala is mainly through Neighborhood Networks along with Government palliative care units. Neighborhood Network in Palliative Care (NNPC) started in 1999 by large scale community participation in north Kerala (Malabar region). The NNPC has recognized as the model for developing countries by WHO. Four agencies were actively involved in building up the NNPC in Kerala, which are

- Malappuram initiative in palliative care

- Pain and palliative care society, Calicut

- Alpha charitable society, Trissur

5

- Justice Sivaram foundation.

The objectives of NNPC is,

- Empowerment of local community to look after the bed ridden in their area

- To develop a cost effective method for the provision of palliative care.

NNPC includes volunteers in the community and trained professionals. Volunteers are anyone who wants to contribute in the efforts to reduce the suffering of people with illness. Structured training given and trained volunteers encouraged to spend at least two hours per week in helping NNPC activities. Volunteers only plan, organize and administrate the palliative care services in their community. That is, the program is completely 'community owned'. The medical doctors and nurses who got training in palliative care they help the volunteers to give medical and nursing care to the needy people.

In Kozhikode district, today there are fifty one (51) NNPC units are working. It is the district where more number of NNPC units is working successfully. To evolve such a program and become most success in this district there are lot of factors were there, that enabled and carrying on this program successfully. We can call those factors as "enabling factors for Neighbourhood Network in Palliative Care (NNPC)". The encyclopaedia of public health describes enabling factors as the factors that makes it possible (easier) for individuals or population to change their behaviour or the environment. And oxford bibliography define enabling factors as "component of combination following forces that are take place together, influence the degree of initiation and continuation of some type of action." . So there is a scope to study about the enabling factors of NNPC. In other sense identifying enabling factors is nothing but it is studying the program itself. Few substantive studies and documentation on the enabling factors of NNPC in Malabar region, hence this study conducted with the objective of understanding factors that enabled the implementation and successful running of NNPC in the district of Kozhikode. Kozhikode District is a district of Kerala state, by the 2011 census there are four taluks, twelve block panchayats and 78 panchayats. And the total population is 3,086,293. And the number of NNPC units is 51, that is majority of panchayats have one NNPC unit. The panchayats does not have NNPC unit is getting services from

6

the surrounding panchayat's NNPC unit, that means the coverage of palliative care service is comparatively high in Kozhikode district.

## RATIONAL FOR THE STUDY, AIM AND OBJECTIVES

The present study was undertaken to explore the enabling factors for the program called Neighbourhood Network in Palliative Care (NNPC) in Kozhikode district of Kerala. As part of the study, maximum possible factors are documented that have helped the implementation and promotion of worldwide recognized palliative care model, NNPC. When we identify and understand the enabling factors of any successful program then it will be easy to replicate the same program into other geographical areas according to the need of the particular contexts.

### Aim

The main aim of the study was to work towards orienting the need of palliative care service provision for the needy population in India. It is also an attempt to explore the factors that are contributed to the success of a community owned health program in a third world country.

### Objective

- To explore the enabling factors that made NNPC happened/happening in Kozhikode district of Kerala

# METHODOLOGY

## Study site

The study was conducted in Kozhikode district, Kerala, India. By the 2011 census total population of the district is 3,086,293. And district contains four taluks, twelve block panchayats and 78 panchayats. The number of Neighborhood Network in Palliative Care (NNPC) units is 51.

## Study Subjects

In-depth Interview (IDI) conducted with 11 study participants from various stakeholders to explore different types of enabling factors for Neighborhood Network in Palliative Care (NNPC).

Stakeholders are:-

1) Pain and Palliative Care Society (PPCS) and Institute of Palliative Medicine (IPM), Calicut.

Neighborhood Network in Palliative Care (NNPC) formed in 1999 jointly by four organizations, PPCS was one among from those four organizations. Pain and Palliative Care Society (PPCS) is a right based Civil Society Organization for people living with incurable and debilitating illness. Formed in 1993, they are the first charitable society for community based palliative care in Low and Middle income countries. PPCS has the distinction of initiating the first community volunteer program and the first home care program for the bedridden patients to its credit. Later in 2001 PPCS launched Institute of Palliative Medicine (IPM) and it became nodal center for NNPC activities in the region.

2) Community Based Organizations.

In the state of Kerala, at present there are around 200 palliative care units. In Kozhikode district it is 51. Majority of them are organized and supported by Community Based Organizations (CBO). Most of them are independent units, but some are based in government and private hospitals. The CBOs are mostly supported by local communities, are self-sustainable in terms of manpower, money and other amenities and dependent on trained volunteers for organizing the services and psychosocial support.

3) Civil society organizations.

Civil society has played crucial role in the development and determination of palliative care services in the region. It includes political parties, religious organizations and charities. Media also have an important role.

4) Beneficiaries:

The patients and families benefit directly from the services. The local community also benefits through enhancement of social capital, improving skills and confidence and the process of empowerment.

## Ethics

The Institutional Ethics Committee (IEC) of University of Hyderabad, Hyderabad approved the study protocol and methods. Information and purpose of the study was discussed with the participants and cleared their doubts about the study.

## Study Method

The selection of participants was purposive. The respondents were identified and then done in-depth interviews to explore the enabling factors that made NNPC happened/happening in Kozhikode district of Kerala. All interviews were recorded as audio files and interviews were in Malayalam. An interview guideline was prepared and listed the questions to be asked. In addition literature search was done to understand about the program in detail. Later Qualitative analysis was done, audios transcribed and translated into English. And output is presented as thematic analysis.

## Study Instrument

In-depth interview was used to collect data about the enabling factors for Neighborhood Network in Palliative Care in Kozhikode district of Kerala. In-depth interviews with different stakeholders helped to explore the different aspects of the program

## Literature review

**Palliative Care**

*Understanding palliative care begins with the story of hospice. 'Hospice' comes from a Latin word* Hospitium, *meaning hospitality, and was used in the middle Ages in Europe and Mediterranean regions to describe a place of rest for travelers and pilgrims. Established and run by religious orders, these places offered special hospitality and care to travelers who were far from home and to people who were ill or dying. The hospice disappeared for a while, but re-emerged in the 19th century in the UK and France particularly, again run by religious orders, and again caring for people who were terminally ill, but also providing accommodation for the incurable and destitute* (http://en.wikipedia.org/wiki/Palliative_care#History)

The modern use of the term hospice dates from 1967 with the opening of St Christopher's Hospice, London, established by Dr Cicely Saunders, later Dame Cicely Saunders (1918 – 2005). At that time there was a growing awareness that 20th century medical advances, while offering a cure for many illnesses, also resulted in the health system ignoring those people who could not be cured. Cicely Saunders, originally a nurse, then a social worker (almoner), finally studied medicine to meet this challenge, the neglect of the suffering of the terminally ill. Her work in building St Christopher's Hospice and her approach to pain and symptom management, recognizing the multi-dimensional nature of suffering and the need for emotional, psychological and spiritual support for both the terminally ill patient and their family was the foundation for modern hospice and palliative care practice (http://www.pallcare.asn.au/about/history-of-palliative-care/late-20th-century-palliative-care).

The term 'palliative care' was first used in 1975 by Canadian surgeon Balfour Mount, an early Saunders pupil. Returning to French speaking Quebec, he needed to avoid the word hospice because of the poor reputation, particularly the connotation of destitution, associated with these institutions in France. Mount developed a comprehensive hospital-based service at the Royal Victoria Hospital, Montreal that included an in-patient ward, consultation service, home care program, and bereavement support service under the name Palliative Care service by which he meant non-curative therapy aimed at improving the quality of life (http://www.medscape.com/viewarticle/707801_2).

Palliative care was first introduced in 1990 by the World Health Organization (WHO) (2004) and is currently defined as "an approach to care which improves quality of life of patients and their families facing life-threatening illness through prevention, assessment, and treatment of pain and other physical, psychological, and spiritual problems." WHO (2004) further describes palliative care for children as the active total care of the child's body, mind, and spirit, as well as a means of providing support to the family. The goals of palliative care can be summarized as providing relief from suffering, pain and other distressing symptoms, psychological, emotional and spiritual care and creation of a support system that helps the individual to live as actively as possible (Mudigonda & Mudigonda 2010, Walsh et al. 1994).

Simply put, it can be said that the aim (Albers et al. 2010) of any palliative care program is to improve the quality of life of patients to the maximum. The term "palliative care" implies a personalized form of health care. It extends the healthcare professional's mandate beyond the biomedical model to the wider horizon necessary if one is to attend to suffering as well as the biology of disease, caring as well as curing, quality of life as well as quantity of life. The patient and family or significant others are taken together as the unit of care in assessment of needs related to illness. The aim of palliative care is to support optimal quality of life and to foster healing— that is, a shift in response towards an experience of integrity and wholeness on the continuum of the quality of life (Balfour Mount, Geoffrey Hanks, Lorna McGoldrick. 1998).

**Modes of Palliative Care (PC) delivery**

The social, cultural and political context determines how palliative care can be delivered (Casadio et al. 2010). Palliative care provided by a specialized palliative care team or institution-based palliative care like hospice care has been documented (Hearn & Higginson 1998, Tierney et al. 1998) to improve quality of life of terminally ill cancer patients in high income countries. However, these will not be readily transferrable to situations that exist in low and middle income countries where human, technical and financial resources are in short supply. Despite 20 years of existence, national palliative care coverage remains under two percent (Sallnow,

Kumar & Numpeli 2010). A report from "The Economist" Intelligence Unit (2010) ranking 40 countries across the world on "Quality of Death Index" based on 24 indicators, put India (score of 1.9 out of 10) at the bottom. The same report mentions that the State of Kerala, if assessed on the same measures, would rank among the top. Kerala provides two thirds of India's existing palliative care services (Paleri & Numpeli 2005) through a more realistic model of home based care (Stjernsward 2005).

**Neighborhood Network in Palliative Care (NNPC)**

In line with the Alma-Ata Declaration and based on the principle that it is the duty of the healthy in the society to take care of the ill, the Neighborhood Network in Palliative Care (NNPC) formed in 2001, called upon the local community to take responsibility for the care of the terminally ill in their midst (Sallnow, Kumar & Numpeli 2010). Volunteers willing to spare two hours a week to care for the sick in their community are given structured training to identify the problems of the chronically ill and to organize effective interventions. A network of trained doctors and nurses provide technical support to the community volunteers.

NNPC has grown rapidly and now caters to the care needs of more than 2500 patients every week, 30 percent of whom are cancer patients (Sallnow, Kumar & Numpeli 2010). Palliative care is an effective intervention for meeting the care needs of people at the end of their lives (WHO 2002).

The attempt by NNPC was 'to develop a sustainable community owned service capable of offering comprehensive long term care and palliative care to most of the needy' (Kumar 2007). With the adoption of community-owned home-based palliative care services as the main mode of palliative care (Mudigonda & Mudigonda 2010) in many parts of the world like the NNPC in Kerala and the Hospice Africa Uganda, Kampala, (Hospice Africa Uganda website) WHO suggested that in countries with poor health infrastructure but strong family support, this model is the best way to achieve quality care with maximum coverage (WHO 2007, 2002. Scientifically valid evidence is essential for policymakers of other states of India and resource-constrained countries to adapt similar models for offering care and support to the incurably ill.

The evolution of NNPC in Kerala can be marked as this way (The evolution of palliative care programs in north Kerala, Anil Paleri, Mathews Numpeli1 2005)

1) A NGO called Pain and Palliative Care Society (PPCS) started at Kozhikode in 1993 by a group of people.

2) An outpatient clinic was setup at the Kozhikode Medical College for cancer patients. It was after making MoU with government of Kerala.

3) First link center was established in 1996 at Manjeri in Malappuram district of Kerala

4) Few more clinics raised nearby places.

It was noticed that the link center at Nilambur in Malappuram district were more successful in terms of coverage and fund raising.

- Volunteers involvement was high

- Volunteers did the responsibility of planning, organizing, fund raising and administrating day to day activities.

- Professionals role is only attend to medical issues and do medical management

- Attending social and financial needs of patients and family become the responsibility of volunteers or volunteers took the responsibility of social aspects of care.

This success leads new initiation, and new groups interested in setting up palliative care services in different places. Volunteers were trained and give support to setup palliative care initiative locally by Institute of Palliative Medicine (IPM).

## RESULTS AND DISCUSSION

The participants in the study contributed sufficient information about their lived experiences and about the program with the researcher in an in-depth interview related to community owned program called Neighbourhood Network in Palliative care (NNPC) . They shared their knowledge, observations and lived experiences that contribute to study in detailed to explore enabling factors for NNPC in Kozhikode district.

A thorough understanding of their responses provides ways to develop several themes that are developed from the data analysis. All the themes such as socio cultural factors, health pattern and demographic factors, behavioural and environmental factors, organizational factors, administrative factors, community Participation/ ownership and other factors. These themes along with their corresponding sub-themes with the particular illustration are discussed below by chapter wise.

### 1. Socio cultural factors

Social scientists and public health scholars have made significant insight on the basic social and cultural structures and processes that influence health and health programs. Social and cultural factors influence a health program from its basic concept to inception, the effectiveness of health program, and access to, availability of, and quality. Social and cultural factors also play a role in shaping perceptions of and responses to the health program.

To evolve and sustain a community owned program called NNPC in Kozhikode district of Kerala, there are lot of socio cultural factors are there, that enabled and carrying on this program successfully. It is related to socio cultural political characteristics of the region. Identified those types of characters are described briefly below.

### Culture of charity

It is noted that this region has its own special mechanisms to help people in need by collective efforts. NNPC or palliative care activity consider as one kind of those charity activity. One of respondents (NNPC Volunteer) states that "collective efforts are very common in our society, but in health through palliative care activities we could establish an organized system to help needy people." So through NNPC activities people especially volunteer gets a satisfaction of doing charity. Another volunteer respond like this "in a week two or three days will reserve for palliative care activities, mainly for home care. After that when we came back home will feel so fresh and will get nice peaceful sleep"

In this region we can find other collective efforts for health, example is. In every villages and town there will be lot of charity organizations. They raise fund for treatment of poor people and distribute medical equipment for those who needed and not affordable that. Another aspect of charity is that in almost every day in Malayalam newspapers we can find the ads or news for collecting contributions for the treatment of poor people. These efforts are initiating locally by collective of local people. Through this kind of activities thousands of economically backward people are getting benefits. So this culture of charity enhanced the initiation of palliative care activities in the region.

**History of successful community owned program**

'Panapayatt' is a system of money exchange existing in the region. This can call as community owned program in financing. It is a kind of get together, usually condected by a person who need money for some purpose of his life. The person invites all his friends, neighbors and knowing people to come his house or any particular venue, where this organized. On the day tea and some snacks are arranged to the invitees. The guests are supposed to give some amount of money to the host and it is recorded in register

At the end of the day host who conducting 'panapayatt' gets huge amount of money by summing up all those little cash given by hundreds of people who attended the party. The objective of 'panapayatt' is to offer financial help to people. The money one receives is supposed to be given to those who gave him, on the day conduct 'panapayatt'. When one needs little huge money for any purpose, he conducts 'panapayatt' and uses the money he gets. This system of money exchange can be seen in most of the part of Kozhikode district.

One of respondent puts his argument in this way "the collective efforts are nothing but it is the continuation of our cultural history. That is, in financing we have our own mechanism 'panapayatt'. It has been exist in our society from long back. Like this palliative care activity is a community owned mechanism in health care provision." That means the cultural history of the region is very favorable for community owned programs. Another examples of community owned initiatives are many successful self-help groups, which are very active in the region.

## 2. Disease pattern and demographic factors

There are lots of incurable and long term diseases are very much prevalent in the region as like any other geographical area. That includes stroke, spinal cord injuries, cancer, mental disorders, old age problems, diabetes, blood pressure, heart diseases, lung problems, kidney disorders and AIDS. Cancer patients were traditionally viewed as the primary recipients of palliative care, but it is increasingly recognized that good end of life care is important in the management of patients with any incurable disease, whatever the diagnosis (dementia, chronic chest or heart disease, Parkinson's disease, frail older people with several long term conditions).

Society realized that the care of this terminally ill people is the responsibility of community. The problems or difficulties of terminally ill patients cannot solve by a doctor or hospital alone. In fact conventional health system can do only very least for the terminally ill patients. So NNPC raised as a mechanism to provide care for most unprivileged sections in the community, that is terminally ill people, old people and disabled. One respondent explains about the situation of NNPC has started in that panchayat "in our area there are lot of people are there with incurable diseases. Many cancer patients are there. Lot of people died with cancer. There is a rubber plantation in this panchayat, there used to aerial spraying of pesticides by helicopter. That leads to high prevalence of cancer in this area. That time we did not have electricity and phone but helicopter comes in every month that was a wonder for us that time. But now we are facing with lot of incurable health problems because of that aerial spraying of pesticides. Only in this panchayat more than 300 people are under treatment for cancer now. This is registered cases, actual number will be more. In fact what made NNPC active in this area is that, people are facing lot of health problem they are very known people may be relatives or friends. Need to do something for them that made NNPC active in the area"

Another important factor is that due to demographic transition, old age people number is increasing in our society day by day. They will be having health problems related to aging. They need continuous care. but in home people are not available to take care their old people. At this juncture local community has taken the responsibility of caring old age people in the locality through NNPC activities.

## 3. Behavioural and environmental factors

### Vibrant civil and political society

Identifying the health priorities and social behavioural and environmental determinants is having lot of importance in any program implementation. Kerala society is generally well known as its vibrant civil and political nature. In case of NNPC also we can clearly notice that the nature of society have geared the program implementation and leads to great success. At the beginning majority of volunteers was retired employees, mainly school teachers and other government employees. One of the participants clearly states that "at the early stage, lot of retired people came to palliative care activities. They have decided their remaining life for charity and social services. Young people were very less at that time." It means the vibrant political and civil natures of society have helped the implementation of NNPC in the region.

Another interesting fact is that, lot of people have fed up with conventional political activities of established political parties. They are seeking this NNPC activities are new platform for them. Another volunteer responds like this "now a days political parties are facing problem in getting people for their activities at local level, the number of people who goes to rally and shout 'zindabad' are reduced" so lot of young and active people are now working with NNPC units at local level. The NNPC unit gives them a platform for social activities.

### Extensive newspaper audience

Kerala has highest newspaper consumption per capita of any state in India according to many reports. This habit of newspaper reading in every morning makes people aware of lot of things happening around the world. The information and awareness about the palliative care activities also circulated widely through newspapers in the region. 'Malayala Manorama' a Malayalam newspaper had given a feature on palliative care movement in 2008. And another Malayalam newspaper 'Madhyamam' has its own initiative for helping economically backward patients. The project of 'Mahyamam' is called 'Santhwanam'. Another fact is that we can see separate section for charity news in Malayalam newspapers. When I asked to some old volunteers about how they got information about palliative care activities they all were given same answer "through newspaper".

**Good transport facilities in the villages**

It is another factor, transport facilities in the villages have helped/helping to render palliative care services in each and every corner of the villages. Every palliative care unit in the district has their own vehicles to go for home care. So the transport facilities in the villages is the another factor of success of palliative care movement in the region. One of the respondents says "whenever anyone needs any help from palliative care unit, what they need to do is that just give a call to the palliative care unit. We will go to the home where patient is there in our vehicle with a nurse and one or two volunteers"

## 4. Organizational factors

### Institute of Palliative Medicine (IPM)

Institute of Palliative Medicine is located in the Medical College campus, Kozhikode, Kerala, India. It started in 2004. The Institute was designated as W.H.O collaboration center in October 2010. In north Malabar region IPM works as nodal agency. It gives structured training for volunteers, doctors and nurses. And IPM supports volunteers to initiate palliative care activities locally by helping them to start NNPC unit in their locality. After starting the NNPC unit in locality IPM continuously assists them to build capacity by further training for volunteers and staffs. One volunteer tells his experience like this "I got information about the palliative care volunteers training camp by newspaper, so I attended that training camp along with one of my friend. It was four days camp in Calicut Christian College, Kozhikode. It was conducted by IPM Calicut. After that camp only we have setup a palliative care unit here." IPM also runs an outpatient unit, inpatient unit and home care unit along with its active research work in palliative care medicine. So IPM has an important role in palliative care movement in the region.

### Kozhikode Initiative in Palliative care (KIP)

It is a coordination committee of all NNPC units in the Kozhikode district.it started in 2004. There are 51 palliative care units are there under KIP now. One of KIP official describe about their activity like this "the main duty which KIP has doing now is, it find out doctors and nurses who are willing to work with NNPC and connect them with NNPC units. Another important work is that giving training to the volunteers and volunteer's trainees. It also acts as the middle agent between government and NNPC units by collecting fund and medicines from government machineries and distributing that to the NNPC units in the district". Along with this activities IPM do more things in terms of arranging meeting in every month for one representative from each palliative care units. In meeting every representative read their unit report. Report includes the activities that particular unit done in previous month and number of people who got benefit with that unit in previous month. If any unit has done any innovative activity that will get know for other units, if needed they can use that thing. So the meeting will help to share and discuss about new ideas and activities doing by any NNPC unit. KIP conducts various programs to raise awareness in the population. One NNPC volunteer tells like this "we need to document each activity which our unit has doing. Every month unit meeting will be there, in that meeting need to read the report and later that we need do report in district meeting." So KIP monitor each NNPC unit's activity and give technical support to improve their unit level performance.

## 5. Administrative factors

### A) Collaboration with local community groups

**Clubs**: - we can notice that local clubs are there in every village in the district. This clubs are generally collective of youths in that locality. They will be having a place in that locality to get-together all of its members. Most of the clubs will be having permanent spaces like office kind of things for gathering. This clubs are actually works as a hanging out point or entertainment spot for youths in the locality. Evenings they gather there and play or do something. Usually newspapers and magazines will be available at this place. Other than this entertainment act they do social service activities also like conducting different programs in the community with collaborating outside agencies. Example is, local clubs conduct blood donation camp, organ donation awareness programs, health camps etc with the help of other agencies or organizations.

One respondent states "our NNPC is having very strong relation with many clubs and self-help groups in this panchayat; our many volunteers are active members of this clubs, mainly youth volunteers. And local clubs also help NNPC to raise fund in the locality." So how this local clubs plays role in NNPC is that, they supply their members to the NNPC unit as volunteers in palliative care activities and they actively participate in the fund raising process of NNPC unit. Many clubs do separate fund raising through their activity and donate that amount to the NNPC unit or utilize the amount for the care of economically backward patient in that locality. One NNPC volunteer and he is also an active member of local club says "when we need any driver urgently for palliative care unit and the registered volunteers are not available to drive, I call my friends in the club and anyone of them will come" this are the clear examples of how local clubs are collaborating with NNPC units in different ways.

**Self-help groups**:- Local self-Help Groups (SHG) are registered or unregistered groups of micro entrepreneurs having homogenous social and economic backgrounds, voluntarily coming together to save regular small sums of money, mutually agreeing to contribute to a common fund and to meet their emergency needs on the basis of mutual help. The group members use collective wisdom and peer pressure to ensure proper end-use of credit and timely repayment. This system eliminates the need for collateral and is closely related to that of solidarity lending, widely used by microfinance institutions. To make the book-keeping simple enough to be handled by the members, flat interest rates are used for most loan calculations (Wikipedia). Usually in self-help groups members will be so closed each other. As the same way clubs are interacting with NNPC unit self-help groups also act.

**Kudumbashree**:- Kudumbashree means 'prosperity of the family'. It is a state-sponsored, self-help organization for women aiming to empower, educate and reduce poverty. It started in Alappuzha in 1993 and a project in Malappuram followed quickly. The Government of Kerala scaled up the project in 1998 to cover the state as a whole and set the target of alleviating poverty by 2008. Each village has a branch where women form 'Neighborhood Groups' comprised of 20–45 families. They design plans for poverty relief, education and improvement in female and child health. The Neighborhood Kudumbashree group then facilitates their training and provides loans and support for the setting up of 'micro-enterprises' such as soap and basket making. The organization provides the support for the initial development of the venture, but the women subsequently run the business independently. Health awareness is an important aspect of Kudumbashree. The coordinators of the NNPC met with those running Kudumbashree at state level and discussed the possibility of collaboration. Subsequently, talks about the NNPC and palliative care were given at the meetings, and those interested became volunteers. Today a large number of the volunteers in NNPC come from Kudumbashree and indeed they are now fully responsible for running a number of palliative care units (The role of religious, social and political groups in Palliative care in Northern Kerala, Libby Sallnow and Shabeer Chenganakkattil 2005). In Kozhikode district also Kudumbashree works strongly. Every ward in a panchayat has one or two Kudumbashree units; sometimes it is more in number. One respondent says "In our NNPC unit volunteers are there from different political parties and religions. Most of our female volunteers are from different Kudumbasree units in the panchayat. Earlier in our NNPC we did not have any female volunteers. Nurse was the only female presence". Female volunteers are very essential in every NNPC units. Because female patients are registered under NNPC need supportive care, sometimes female volunteers only can provide that sort of services in proper way. So the collaboration with Kudumbashree made NNPC activities more comprehensive and effective by female participation in palliative care activity.

**B) Collaboration with educational institutions**

Student participation is an important aspect of NNPC. 'Students in Palliative Care' is an initiative by the young, vibrant student community of Kozhikode city. The organization on since January 2010 is aimed at organizing adequate and affordable support programs for the bed ridden, the incurably ill and the dying people. SIPC, since its inception has been instrumental in ensuring consistent involvement of students in spreading awareness on palliative care, hands on patient care and mobilizing volunteers, material and financial resources (http://www.instituteofpalliativemedicine.org). One of NNPC volunteer explains how locally students are participating, "we conducted a camp for students with the collaboration of nearby educational institutes. About 120 students participated in that camp, it was two day camp. In that we gave the foundation of palliative care. The program was sponsored by Kozhikode Initiative in Palliative care (KIP). After that the students who have participated in that camp comes for our home care visit and they help us in fund raising programs also" some colleges in the districts have palliative care volunteers units in the college, they work with nearby NNPC unit.

## 6. Community participation/ownership

**Volunteer**

Community participation can be loosely defined as the involvement of people in a community to solve their own problems (IPM 2010). It is a very broad concept and in the context of a program, it can mean anything from simple feedback from the community to major involvement in all the phases and areas of the program. NNPC run with community participation. An ownership of the program with participation of the local community in the need assessment, planning, implementation, resource mobilization, day to day management and evaluation of the program is community volunteer. It may not be possible for each and every member of the affected population to contribute to a program equally but attempts can be made to actively involve as many key groups and individuals as possible.

Community volunteers play a major role in the program. Their activities related to the care of the patient and family need to be supported by health care professionals at various levels. One NNPC volunteer explain about volunteering " we, most of volunteers now working with NNPC became NNPC volunteer by participating volunteer camp conducted by IPM. Volunteer do lot of things like, planning and administrate palliative care activity in unit, fund raise for the initiative and we arrange food for starving family, spending time with a lonely patient, mobilizing support for the patient and family from the community, offering emotional support to the patient and families etc"

We can categorize volunteers into two groups, untrained volunteer and trained volunteer. Untrained volunteers are who are cooperating with local NNPC unit and they did not get intensive training in palliative care formally. They help NNPC units to collect food for patients, for transport like drivers and to raise fund. Such volunteers can be motivated by several sensitization and awareness programs in the community. Student in palliative care mostly work as untrained volunteers. They took the responsibility of such activities (IPM 2010).

Trained Volunteers are who went through intensive training program. They are able to provide patient care in many ways like emotional support, basic nursing activities and help with mobility. They only taking and doing home care with the help of professionals. And look after the social and economic need of patients. Apart from

25

this responsibility community volunteers do organizational and administration of services. Examples include Regular awareness program in the community, Training the family members to look after the patient, Training volunteers in the community, Administrative management of the unit and fund raising.

**Micro fund raising**

Community ownership of the program usually ensures good financial support from the community. Community participation can include finance generating activities and this may be a key starting point in giving communities greater responsibility, removing dependence on external support and promoting sustainability. It is in the form of donation boxes at public places and shops, collections from student community, donations of cash and kind during festive occasions etc. and people contribute money to the NNPC units as like contributing to the holy places in regular basis.

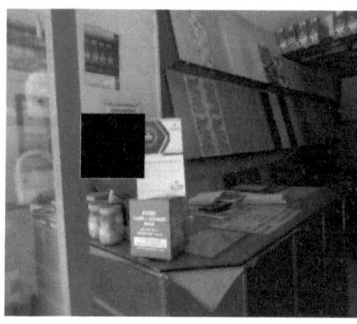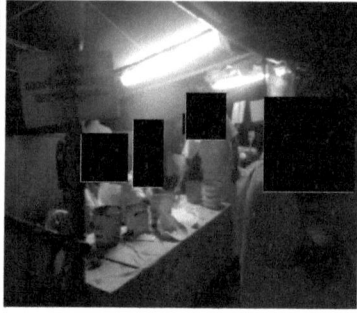

First picture showing a box at shop to collect money for NNPC unit in that locality, Second one is the picture from a temple festival in a village in Kozhikode district there local NNPC unit have kept a stall for collecting money for NNPC unit.

One of NNPC volunteers tells about fund raising ""75% of our money came as donations of less than fifty rupees. We keep boxes in all shops, homes and public places". So through this micro fund raising process NNPC could make awareness in the community is that, this program is our own for us and that leads more community participation and success of the program.

## 7. Support from civil society organizations, religious groups and political parties

In a retrospective paper titled 'The role of religious, social and political groups in Palliative care in Northern Kerala' by Libby Sallnow and Shabeer Chengunakkatil traces the roots of collaboration of different groups with Palliative care movement in Kerala. The first community based palliative care unit started by a doctor in Manjeri, Malappuram district. He was part of a Muslim religious group Called Kerala Naduvathul Mujaahid (KNM). This religious organization has taken up the initiative of starting palliative care units in different part of northern Kerala, especially in Malappuram and Kozhikode district. The second community palliative care unit was started by a Hindu religious group in Wayanad. Christian religious groups also were very active in palliative care services. In Kozhikode district there was a palliative care training center and palliative care inpatient unit, this was set up by Medical Sisters of St. Joseph. Many other groups also like local units of political parties and merchant associations also involved in palliative activities at different level.

One of the NNPC volunteer tells about his unit "it was started in 2008, the people who were behind this unit was some Muslim League people. But at the time of initiation itself they have included all party cadres in the unit. Now our unit members constitute all most all political party members" it is the interesting fact about the palliative care movement in the district, that no groups which have took the initiation of starting up NNPC unit locally did not try to patronize the unit. They have ensured all community participation and rendered services to everyone in that locality. Actually when a NNPC unit established in a locality, then it became under the whole community in that location for the people who are living that locality.

The civil society organizations play a crucial role in fund raising for NNPC units. They are actively involved in the process of fund raising in different ways. Example is that, one respondent tells "local groups like clubs and self-help groups generously contribute to us. They help us to reach each and every house in the panchayat, local club members go to each houses and collect money from the boxes which they have already given to the household. And they give that to NNPC unit" another volunteers says "we collect more amount of money in the month of Ramadan, that time in mosque after prayers collect money for palliative care. People contribute largely that time." Ramadan is the month in Arabic calendar, when Muslims observe this as a month of fasting. Charity is very important during Ramadan, which called as Zakat. So during Ramadan people contribute more money toward charity activities. Palliative care activities are getting a huge amount of money during the month of Ramadan.

The support of various groups makes NNPC as successful model for community owned program in palliative care.

## 8. Package of services

The range of services is providing through a community based palliative care program are very much in line with the concept of total care in palliative care. Home care is the mainstay of these services. The home care team consisting of health care professionals and community volunteers visit the patient and family at home, discuss the problems and offer appropriate services. Development of the wider network of community volunteers in the neighbourhood helps ensures continuity of services between home visits and also the necessary social support for the patient and family. The following diseases are carefully following by NNPC; it includes stroke, spinal cord injuries, cancer, mental disorders, old age problems, diabetes, blood pressure, heart diseases, lung problems, kidney disorders and AIDS.

Nurse led home care services are the main stay of home care services. Nurses in the team can address the nursing needs, help the community volunteers in offering emotional support, ensure proper documentation and seek support from the doctor in the team in handling other physical problems. A doctor with necessary training in palliative care plays the major supportive role for the home care team. The doctor offers advice and consultations and makes home visits when suggested by the home care team. Very often, the doctor is part of the team that maintains the palliative care outpatient clinic or inpatient unit. This person may be the local general practitioner or any their doctor, provided they have had their training in palliative care.

Community Volunteers are the backbone of home care programs. Volunteers, as mentioned earlier, depending on their training, skills and experience, they offer a variety of services to the patients and families. These include, Emotional support, Basic nursing, Follow up of professional home care, Linking up with the professional team, Social support to the affected family by way of, Food for the family,

Educational support for children, Helping with transport to hospital, Linking with other support groups, Helping to make potential benefits from government / NGOs available, Rehabilitation.

In rehabilitation, mainly focuses on disabled persons. Those who are on bedridden for a long time, for them a special program is under NNPC. This program is called 'footprints'. It is for empowering people who are in bedridden for a long time by training them to make small handlooms work like making detergent powder, umbrella, ornaments etc. those products are marketing in the community by using the network of NNPC. This partially supported by Sir Ratan Tata Trust (IPM).

One of NNPC volunteer narrates the tune of variety services which they are doing "when we go for home care, we sit with the patient. Patients will tell whatever things they wanted to tell. Family members tell whatever they want to tell. Economic crisis, difficulties, like that many things. They will tell and we will listen carefully. After hearing we will seek the solutions for the difficulties. If food is not available we will arrange that or if medicine is needed we will provide that. If anything else they want, that. Sometimes we make bath patient. We will change dress. If they want to go somewhere, in possible cases we will take them to those places"

Apart from this all thing some NNPC units provides physiotherapy facility in the unit for all people in the community. One NNPC nurse tells "from the begging of this year onwards we have arranged physiotherapy facility in our unit. One physiotherapist usually comes in every Wednesday. After one month we had to buy some more equipment because of many number of people are utilizing this" this shows that how effective the range of programs under NNPC.

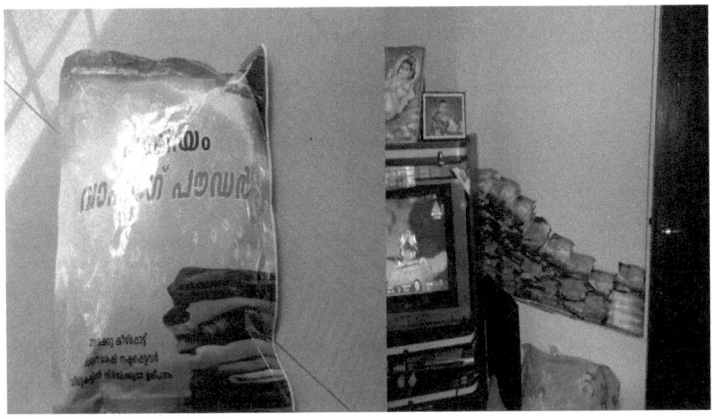

This picture shows the washing powder packets made by person who is disabled from the home. This is facilitated by the local NNPC unit at Edachery in Kozhikode district. This product named as 'Pallium washing powder'. After the production from home NNPC unit collect the products and sell in market. Through this program disabled people get livelihood and thus they become more empowered.

## Conclusion

In the district of Kozhikode, Kerala, at present there are around 51 NNPC units. Majority of them are organized and supported by Community Based Organizations (CBO). Most of them are independent units, but some are based in government and private hospitals. The CBOs are mostly supported by local communities, are self-sustainable in terms of manpower, money and other amenities and dependent on trained volunteers for organizing the services and psychosocial support. In many places, the Local Self Governments Institutions (LSGI) have come forward to work with these groups in providing home visits, outpatient service and free drugs for the poor. Recognizing the need of palliative care as a primary health care and the importance of home care services for patients with long term/ incurable diseases, the Government of Kerala recently brought out a Kerala State Policy for Pain and Palliative Care Services in April 2008. My current study has explored few enabling factors for this community owned palliative care program. These are the few factors which we could identify easily. At the same there might be complex factors which helping the success of the program. Intensive study has to be done to explore maximum enabling factors for Neighborhood Network in Palliative Care.

## Limitations

This study is not without its limitations. The first one was inability to reach and recruit appropriate study participants more in numbers during the field work because of lack of experience and lack of institutional support and the inability to accurately interpret, analyze, and validate data/findings.

## Recommendations

The demonstration of impact of this model of palliative care delivery (NNPC) where the community assumes the responsibility for the total care of the patient, should pave the way for implementation of similar initiatives in other parts of India, which have a dismal palliative coverage of less than two percent.

Public health bodies should take the initiative to start up provision for palliative care services with collaboration of other institutes and interested agencies

Extensive study should be done on NNPC to explore more factors that have contributed the success of the program, to scale up the program.

## References

1. Kumar SK. Kerala, India: a regional community-based palliative care model. J Pain Symptom Manage 2007; 33: 623-27.

2. Mudigonda T, Mudigonda P. Palliative cancer care ethics: principles and challenges in the Indian setting. Indian J Palliat Care 2010; 16: 107-10.

3. Paleri A, Numpeli M. The evolution of palliative care programmes in North Kerala.Indian J Palliat Care 2005; 11: 15-18.

4. Sallnow L, Kumar S, Numpeli M. Home-based palliative care in Kerala, India: the Neighbourhood Network in Palliative Care. Prog Palliat Care 2010; 18: 14-17.

5. Seamark D, Ajithakumari K, Burn G, Saraswathi Devi P, Koshy R, Seamark C. Palliative care in India. J R Soc Med 2000; 93: 292-95.

6. Stjernsward J, Foley KM, Ferris FD. The public health strategy for palliative care. J Pain Symptom Manage 2007; 33: 486-93.

7. Stjernsward J. Community participation in palliative care. Indian J Palliat Care 2005; 11: 111-17.

8. Sureshkumar K, Rajagopal MR. Palliative care in Kerala. Problems at presentation in 440 patients with advanced cancer in a south Indian state. Palliat Med 1996; 10: 293-98.

9. World Health Organisation. Cancer fact sheet No. 297. Geneva: WHO; 2011. Available at www.who.int/mediacentre/factsheets/fs297/en/index.html

10. World Health Organisation. Palliative Care. (Cancer control: knowledge into action: WHO guide for effective programmes; module 5). Geneva: WHO; 2007. Available at http://www.who.int/cancer/media/FINAL-Palliative%20Care%20Module.pdf

11. World Health Organisation. WHO National Cancer Control Programmes: policies and managerial guidelines – 2nd ed. Geneva: WHO; 2002. Available at http://www.who.int/cancer/media/en/408.pdf

12. Human Rights Watch. Global State of Pain Treatment: Access to Medicines and Palliative Care. New York: Human Rights Watch; May 2011. Available from http://www.hrw.org/reports/2011/06/02/global-state-pain-treatment-0

13. Economist Intelligence Unit. The quality of death: Ranking end-of-life care across the world. London: The Economist; 2010. Available at www.eiu.com/sponsor/lienfoundation/qualityofdeath

14. Divya Khosla, Firuza D Patel, Suresh C Sharma. Palliative Care in India: Current Progress and Future Needs. Indian Journal of Palliative Care / Sep-Dec 2012 / Vol-18 / Issue-3.

15. Harmala Gupta. Community participation in palliative care: a comment. Indian J Palliative Care | June 2005 | Vol. 11 | Issue 1.

16. Suresh Kumar, Mathews Numpeli. Neighborhood network in palliative care. Indian J Palliative Care | June 2005 | Vol. 11 | Issue 1.

17. The Hindu newspaper report. Making a DIFFERENCE. Published: October 20, 2012 00:00 IST.

18. Cherian Koshy. The Palliative Care Movement in India: Another Freedom Struggle or a Silent Revolution?. Indian Journal of Palliative Care / Jan-June 2009 / Vol-15 / Issue-1.

19. Libby Sallnow, Shabeer Chenganakkattil. The role of religious, social and political groups in palliative care in Northern Kerala. Indian J Palliative Care | June 2005 | Vol. 11 | Issue 1.

20. Rajashree Chittazhathu, Shamsudeen Moideen. Training community volunteers and professionals in the psychosocial aspects of palliative care. Indian J Palliative Care | June 2005 | Vol. 11 | Issue 1.

21. Institute of palliative medicine. www.instituteofpalliativemedicine.org

**Interview guideline**

In-depth Interview (IDI) will be conducted with the selected participants from various stakeholders to explore different types of enabling factors for Neighborhood Network in Palliative Care (NNPC). General questions which have asked when doing Interview given below, according to response related questions asked to get more details.

1. How did you connect with palliative care activities?
2. How you have initiated palliative care activities in their locality?
3. What are the activities/services now available at local palliative care unit?
4. And how it is going on?
5. What are the collaboration made at local level for the activities?
6. How local community is responding?
7. And participating in palliative care services.
8. How are you raising fund for activities?
9. What is their opinion about palliative care movement in the region?
10. What are the factors that you think that contributed/contributing the success of program?

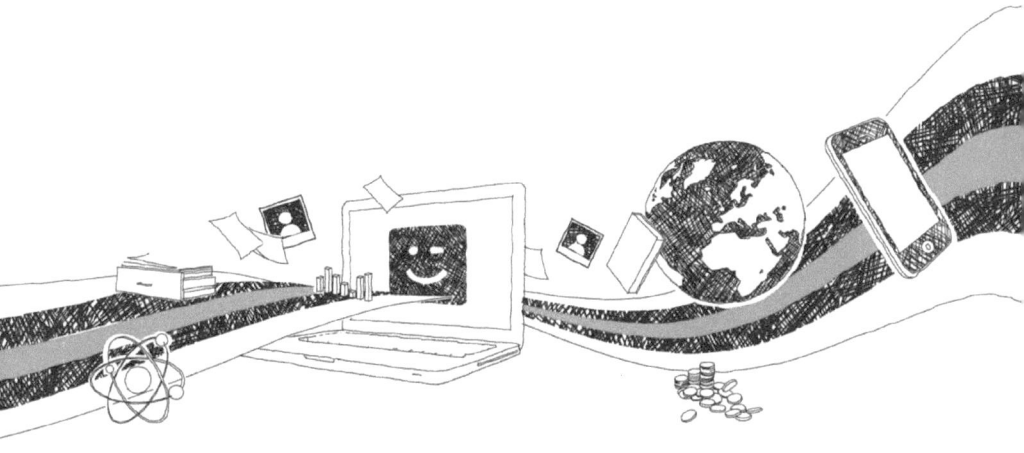
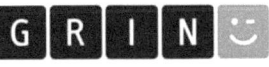